EAT TO BURN YOUR FAT

A Simple 5-Step Strategy to Lose Weight Eating What Your Body Needs

JOSH SIMON

EAT
TO
BURN
YOUR FAT

A Simple 5-Step Strategy to Lose Weight Eating What Your Body Needs

Josh Simon

Table of Contents

Introduction

Did you know that overweight is considered one of the most life-threatening and serious health conditions and has ravaged a great number of Americans, irrespective of age? According to the National Center for Health Statistics, the percentage of adults in the United States aged 20 and above who are obese or overweight ranged from 41.9% in 2017 to 2020. In the same year period, the percentage of adolescents aged 12-19 years who were obese was 22.2%, while the rate of children aged 6-11 years who were obese was 20.7%.

The fact that over 40% of the American population is living with overweight, a condition that not only impacts physical well-being but also weaves its effects into the tapestry of our lives, influencing everything from self-esteem to overall quality of life, is a major cause for concern.

However, this isn't just about numbers. It's about people—individuals striving for a healthier, more vibrant life. And that's where this book comes into play.

Eat to Burn Your Fat: A Simple 5-Step Strategy to Lose Weight Eating What Your Body Needs is not just another diet book or a transitory trend. It's your ally in a comprehensive journey toward sustainable weight loss, better health, and lasting change.

Beyond shedding excess pounds, this book provides you with a deep understanding of the intricacies of metabolism. This biological powerhouse influences how your body burns fat and uses energy. In 10 simple steps, you will learn about the myths and unveiled truths about fat, guiding you through an exploration of healthy eating, exercise, sleep, and stress management.

As you embark on this transformative path, you'll discover not only how to shed those unwanted pounds but also how to reignite your metabolism, bolster your overall health, and embrace a life that is not limited by the scales. Whether you're aiming to drop a dress size or seeking a profound shift in your well-being, this book is your roadmap.

Are you ready to find out the secrets to burn fat while you eat and live a healthier life? Keep reading?

Chapter 1

The Truth About Fat

The topic of fat, more than any other aspect of nutrition and wellness, embodies so much complexity. For far too long, fat has been both villain and savior. But amid this confusion, one thing remains clear—fat is an inescapable, essential element of our existence. It is a part of our biology intertwined with our very survival. So, let's unearth the truth about fat, to separate the myths from the realities, and liberate this complex component of our diets from the shadows of misinformation.

WHAT IS FAT?

Another word for body fat is 'adipose tissue.' It is a natural and necessary component of the human body with multiple functions. It functions as a primary energy storage system, storing surplus calories for later use, as well as providing insulation to regulate body temperature and protect essential organs. Furthermore, adipose tissue produces hormones that affect metabolism and hunger, and it serves as a storage site for fat-soluble vitamins.

DIFFERENT TYPES OF FAT

1. Saturated Fat

Solid fats are another name for saturated fats because they remain stable even when kept at room temperature. These fatty acids have "saturated" carbon structures, meaning that they are filled with hydrogen atoms.

When consumed in large quantities over time, saturated fats may raise health concerns.

Having a diet heavy in saturated fat may cause LDL (low-density lipoprotein) cholesterol levels to rise over time. The likelihood of developing cardiovascular disease or having a stroke increases as a result of this.

NOTE: The following food sources are said to contain saturated fat:

- Processed foods, such as French fries, baked products, and snack foods
- Animal meat and product
- A few vegetable oils, such as cocoa butter, coconut oil, and palm oil
- Dairy products, excluding fat-free varieties

2. Unsaturated Fat

Unsaturated fats are liquid at room temperature and are considered heart-healthy fats. They can be further divided into two types:

1. ***Monounsaturated Fats:*** a type of unsaturated fat that remains liquid at room temperature and becomes solid when chilled. They are known for their heart-healthy properties and can help reduce levels of low-density lipoprotein (LDL) cholesterol, often referred to as "bad" cholesterol. Foods rich in monounsaturated fats include olive oil, avocados, nuts, and seeds, and they are a beneficial component of a balanced diet.

2. ***Polyunsaturated Fats:*** Unlike monounsaturated fats, polyunsaturated fats remain liquid at room temperature and when chilled. They are essential fats because the body can't produce them on its own, and they must be obtained through the diet. Key sources of polyunsaturated fats include fatty fish, such as salmon and mackerel, flaxseeds, walnuts, and various vegetable oils, like corn and soybean oil.

3. Trans Fat

Trans fats are artificially created. They are the result of a procedure that turns liquid vegetable oils into a more solid state by adding hydrogen. Trans fats are also known as partially hydrogenated oils.

Trans fats are unhealthy and not necessary for good health. They cause a decrease in HDL cholesterol and an increase in LDL cholesterol. This raises the danger of type 2 diabetes, heart disease, and stroke.

Food industries discovered trans fats to be cost-effective and easy to use, which led to their rise in popularity. They can enhance the flavor of food and have a lengthy shelf life.

Trans fats are now frequently used in fast-food restaurants and other eateries since they can be reused repeatedly in commercial fryers.

NOTE: The following food sources are said to contain trans-fat:

- Fast food
- Packaged foods
- French fries
- Stick margarine and shortenings
- Baked goods like biscuits, pies, doughnuts
- Crackers, cookies, and pizza dough

Other Types of Fats Found in the Human Body

White Adipose Tissue (WAT)

This type of fat is the most common and is primarily responsible for energy storage. It can be present beneath the skin (subcutaneous fat) as well as around internal organs (visceral fat). Excess visceral fat is linked to a variety of health problems, including heart disease and type 2 diabetes.

Brown Adipose Tissue (BAT)

Brown fat is primarily engaged in thermogenesis or heat generation. It has a high number of mitochondria and aids the body in the burning of calories to produce heat. BAT is more frequent in newborns, but it can be found in adults as well.

Beige Adipose Tissue

Beige fat cells are transitional cells that can change from white to brown fat features. They can aid in energy expenditure and thermogenesis, making them vital in the regulation of body temperature and metabolism.

Subcutaneous Fat

This is the fat that is stored just beneath the skin and is found throughout the body. While excess subcutaneous fat might be unsightly, it is less metabolically active than visceral fat and is associated with less health hazards.

Visceral Fat

Visceral fat covers and protects internal organs such as the liver, kidneys, and intestines. Excess visceral fat has been related to an increased risk of metabolic disorders such as insulin resistance, heart disease, and high blood pressure.

Epicardial Fat

This is a particular form of visceral fat that is located all around the heart. It has been found that having an excessive amount of epicardial fat is linked to an increased risk of developing heart disease.

SIGNS YOU'RE CONSUMING TOO MUCH FAT

Saturated fat, which is prevalent in animal products like meat, eggs, and dairy, should be consumed in moderation, but in excess can be harmful. There are several warning signals your body may be giving you right now if you're consuming too much of it.

1. You put on unexplained weight

One of the primary signs that you're consuming too much fat in a diet is unexplained or gradual weight gain. This is primarily due to the higher calorie density of fats. Excess dietary fat contributes to an elevated caloric intake. When this intake consistently exceeds the body's energy expenditure, the surplus calories are stored as fat, leading to weight gain over time.

2. Your body fat percentage increases

Did you know that regularly monitoring changes in your body fat percentage can be a good indicator of whether or not you're consuming excess fat? Body fat percentage is a more specific metric than overall weight, helping to distinguish between muscle mass and fat mass. An increase in body fat percentage, especially if not attributable to muscle gain, suggests a potential excess of dietary fat. This nuanced approach to tracking body composition provides a more accurate reflection of fat-related changes, allowing for timely adjustments in dietary choices to maintain a healthy balance and support overall well-being.

3. You experience bloating and other digestive discomfort

Excessive consumption of fats, particularly saturated and trans fats, can have adverse effects on digestive health, leading to discomfort, bloating, and indigestion. These types of fats are known to slow down the digestive process, causing delayed emptying of the stomach and potential disruptions in the normal digestive flow. Additionally, high-fat meals can stimulate the production of bile and digestive enzymes, leading to feelings of fullness, discomfort, and bloating.

4. You feel sluggish and experience low energy levels

Although fat is a crucial energy source for the body, an excessive intake, particularly of unhealthy fats, can result in feelings of sluggishness and low energy levels. Unhealthy fats, such as saturated and trans fats, can contribute to a higher calorie density in the diet, leading to an overabundance of energy that may not be efficiently utilized. This surplus of energy, combined with potential metabolic disruptions, can leave you feeling lethargic and lacking in vitality.

5. You feel pains in your joints

Obesity resulting from an excess accumulation of fat places increased stress on joints, contributing to joint pain and discomfort. The additional weight places a greater load on weight-bearing joints, such as the knees and hips, potentially accelerating wear and tear on the joint tissues. Over time, this increased stress can lead to conditions like osteoarthritis, characterized by inflammation and degradation of joint cartilage.

6. You experience high cholesterol levels

A diet high in unhealthy fats, particularly saturated and trans fats, may contribute to elevated levels of LDL ("bad") cholesterol, heightening the risk of cardiovascular issues. These fats can stimulate the liver to produce more LDL cholesterol, leading to an imbalance in the cholesterol profile. Elevated levels of LDL cholesterol contribute to the formation of plaque in arteries, narrowing them and potentially leading to atherosclerosis, coronary artery disease, and an increased risk of heart attacks and strokes.

Key Takeaways:

In this chapter, we learned:

- What is fat?
- The different types of fat
- Various signs that you're consuming too much fat

In the next chapter, we are going to look at the aspect of metabolism and how it relates to weight management and health.

Chapter 2

The Role of Metabolism in Weight Management

Metabolism, the body's biochemical machinery, is the silent conductor directing how food is turned into energy. This process affects not just our everyday energy levels but also the vital balance of our weight. Those with faster metabolism have higher chances of burning fat compared to those with very low metabolism. So, before we go into the connection between metabolism and weight management, let's first look at what metabolism is in detail.

WHAT IS METABOLISM?

The complex network of biological reactions in the body that transform food into energy is called metabolism. It involves a sequence of chemical processes that release energy necessary for a number of physiological processes by breaking down nutrients in the food we eat.

Metabolism can be broadly categorized into two main components:

- **Catabolism:** This phase involves the breakdown of complex molecules from food, such as carbohydrates, proteins, and fats, into simpler forms. During catabolism, energy is released.

- **Anabolism:** In this phase, the body utilizes the energy released during catabolism to build and synthesize complex molecules, such as proteins and nucleic acids, which are crucial for growth, repair, and maintenance.

HOW METABOLISM WORKS

Metabolism operates as a complex and finely tuned system, orchestrating a series of biochemical processes to convert food into energy and sustain the body's vital functions. The journey begins with the ingestion of food, where macronutrients—carbohydrates, proteins, and fats—are broken down during digestion into their simpler forms: glucose, amino acids, and fatty acids. These building blocks then enter the bloodstream, serving as the raw materials for energy production.

Once in the bloodstream, glucose is readily available for immediate energy use. At the same time, amino acids contribute to protein synthesis and repair. Fatty acids, on the other hand, are either utilized for energy or stored in adipose tissue for later use. Many factors affect this process's efficiency, including the hormonal environment of the body, the activity of enzymes, and the general status of nutrition.

The second phase of metabolism involves cellular respiration, occurring within tiny structures called mitochondria. Here, the derived nutrients undergo oxidation, releasing energy in the form of adenosine triphosphate (ATP). ATP serves as the energy currency for cellular activities, powering essential processes such as muscle contraction, nerve impulse transmission, and maintenance of body temperature. The rate at which these processes occur, known as the metabolic rate, is a key determinant of energy expenditure and, consequently, weight management.

THE CONNECTION BETWEEN METABOLISM AND WEIGHT GAIN

Did you know that there is a complex interplay between metabolism and weight gain? This is influenced by various factors that impact how the body processes and stores energy. Understanding this interplay provides insights into why some individuals may be more prone to weight gain.

Basal Metabolic Rate (BMR)

The Basal Metabolic Rate (BMR), which denotes the energy expended at rest, is a foundational aspect of metabolism and plays a crucial role in weight management. Scientific research has consistently supported the notion that individuals with a lower BMR may burn fewer calories at rest, creating an environment conducive to weight gain when calorie intake exceeds energy expenditure. A study published in the American Journal of Clinical Nutrition (Johnstone et al., 2005) demonstrated the inverse relationship between BMR and the likelihood of weight gain, highlighting that those with a lower BMR may face increased challenges in maintaining a healthy weight due to their inherently lower calorie-burning capacity at rest.

Genetics

Genetic factors significantly shape an individual's metabolic profile, impacting their susceptibility to weight gain. Notably, studies in the field of genetics and metabolism have underscored the heritability of metabolic traits, shedding light on how certain genetic variations can influence the efficiency of calorie utilization. A pioneering study about the intricate relationship between genetics and metabolism led by Speakman and Rance (2008) delved into the genetic regulation of energy expenditure, revealing insights into the intricate relationship between genetics and metabolism. The research emphasized that individuals may inherit specific genetic variations associated with a slower metabolism, creating a predisposition towards increased energy storage and a higher likelihood of weight gain.

In this groundbreaking study, Speakman and Rance (2008) demonstrated that genetic factors play a pivotal role in determining the rate at which the body expends energy. The research involved a comprehensive exploration of metabolic regulation, highlighting the complex interplay between genetic components and energy balance. The results affirmed that individuals with certain genetic predispositions may face challenges in maintaining a healthy weight due to their genetically influenced, inherently slower metabolic rate.

Hormonal Influence

Hormones are like important messengers in the intricate choreography of our body's energy balance and weight control. Think of the thyroid gland as a key player in this hormonal dance floor—it produces hormones that are super important for how our metabolism works. Metabolism is basically how our body uses and burns calories to create energy, and these thyroid hormones are like conductors, guiding this whole process to keep everything in harmony. So, when the thyroid gland is doing its job well, our metabolism dances smoothly, helping us maintain a healthy weight.

In the case of someone with hypothyroidism, it means their thyroid gland isn't as active as it should be, and it produces fewer thyroid hormones. Now, these hormones are like the managers of our body's calorie-burning process or metabolism. So, if there's not enough of them, our body's metabolism slows down. It's like the engine of a car running at a lower speed, making it harder to turn calories into energy efficiently. This slowdown can make it tough for people with hypothyroidism to keep a healthy weight because their bodies aren't burning calories as effectively, leading to weight gain.

Muscle Mass

Lean muscle mass contributes significantly to BMR, as muscle tissue requires more energy at rest than fat tissue. Individuals with lower muscle mass may experience a slower metabolism, making weight gain more likely if dietary habits are not adjusted accordingly.

To simplify this, let's use the illustration of a car. Imagine your body is like a car, and muscles are the engine that burns calories. Now, the more muscle you have, the more calories your body burns, even when you're not doing anything—like when the car engine is running or when the car is parked. This is called your Basal Metabolic Rate (BMR). So, if you have more muscle, your BMR is higher, and you burn more calories at rest. On the other hand, if you have less muscle, it's like having a smaller engine, and your body doesn't burn as many calories when you're just chilling. That's why having less muscle can slow down your metabolism, making it easier to gain weight if you don't adjust how you eat.

So, building and keeping muscles is like giving your body a powerful engine to burn calories. It's not just about looking strong; it helps you keep a healthy weight because your body becomes a more efficient calorie-burning machine, even when you're taking it easy.

Age

Did you know that your metabolism naturally tends to slow down with age? As we get older, our body's calorie-burning engine, also known as metabolism, tends to slow down a bit. Picture it like a car that used to zip around but now cruises at a gentler pace. One reason for this is that we tend to lose some of our muscle mass as we age, and muscles are like the energetic drivers behind our metabolism—they burn calories. Additionally, our hormones, which are like traffic directors telling the body what to do, also go through changes. This natural slowdown in metabolism with age means our body isn't burning calories as quickly, making it easier to gain weight if we keep eating the same way and don't stay active.

Diet and Lifestyle

Let's break down how our eating habits and lifestyle choices can affect our body's calorie-burning engine or metabolism.

Imagine your body is like a well-oiled machine, and the fuel you put in is what keeps it running smoothly. Now, suppose we regularly fill it up with processed foods, sugary snacks, and unhealthy fats. In that case, it's like putting low-quality fuel in the machine. This can mess with how our body processes the calories and can lead to some issues.

One problem is insulin resistance, which is like the machine not responding well to the fuel. When this happens, our body struggles to use the calories effectively, and they end up getting stored as fat instead. It's like the machine starts storing extra fuel in the garage because it can't use it properly. So, if we make poor food choices and don't move around much, it's like not giving our body the right fuel and not using up the stored fuel, which can contribute to gaining weight. It's all about giving our body the good stuff and keeping it active to keep the machine running smoothly.

Key Takeaways:

This chapter has been able to explore the following:

- What is metabolism?
- How metabolism works
- The connection between metabolism and weight gain

Now that we know how metabolism functions and its connection with weight gain, in the next chapter, let's look at why diets often fail despite your efforts to lose weight.

Chapter 3

Why Diets Often Fail

Every time someone diets, they put on an average of 11 pounds. Worse still, they lose both muscle and fat along with weight. They put on much too much fat when they eat again. Their metabolism is slowed down even further than it was before they began dieting, as muscle consumes seven times as many calories as fat. The terrifying fact is that they will require even fewer calories as we advance to stay the same weight.

Surely, you must have met an obese person who insisted they didn't actually consume that much food. They may be telling the truth. Their metabolism is now permanently affected due to their yo-yo dieting habits.

There are just two basic requirements for successful weight loss and maintenance. Instead of trying to force yourself to eat less by restricting your food intake, you should focus on balancing the hormones and brain chemistry that are responsible for hunger and overeating.

The second is to speed up your metabolism naturally, resulting in increased calorie expenditure throughout the day. Sadly, most diets have the reverse effect, making people hungrier and sluggish.

Let's now look at some technical reasons diets often fail:

REASONS DIETS OFTEN FAIL

Inadequate Protein Intake

While there are many acclaimed quick fixes for weight loss, such as fad diets and medications, a healthy diet is the best way to keep the weight off for good. Increasing your protein intake while decreasing your carbohydrate intake is a good place to start. Even though they vary from person to person, the macronutrients you consume still need to be in harmony with one another.

When it comes to weight loss, dietary proteins are more concerned with reducing fat mass than they are with reducing lean body mass. They make you feel fuller for longer and aid in muscle preservation.

A study conducted by the National Library of Medicine found that visceral fat, which may lead to obesity and other health issues, was reduced in older men who consumed more protein. Protein is important for weight control and muscle maintenance, and so is regular, moderate exercise.

Consuming more protein will help you feel full longer and reduce your need to eat every two hours.

Too Much Emphasis on Calories

Calorie counting is an annoying and time-consuming task. Although cutting calories is necessary for weight loss, getting enough of the nutrients your body requires to function optimally is of far greater importance. Calorie counting is important, but it shouldn't be your only criterion for choosing what to eat.

Don't worry too much about how many calories something has and more about what's in it. Think about how quality matters more than quantity. Can you get the same nutritional value from sugar-free, low-calorie Jell-O as you would from low-fat yogurt? Obviously, you can't!

In a similar vein, when you don't consume enough calories, you lose muscle mass rather than fat. It occurs because your body goes into hunger mode and stores fat. In addition to making it more difficult to shed pounds, reducing muscle mass (lean body mass) slows down your metabolism.

Too much calorie restriction can make it hard to maintain your workout routine. In addition, it may cause binge eating at the end of the day. Cutting off sugary drinks and other sources of empty calories will help you shed pounds and feel better in no time.

Not Minding What You Eat

A lot of you see food as more than just something you eat to keep you alive. It can be a source of solace, a method of commemorating milestones, and an expression of affection. Even so, many people regularly resort to eating as a means of relieving stress, boredom, or other unpleasant emotions. All of these factors can contribute to "mindless eating," the practice of eating a lot of food without paying attention to or enjoying it. This might be detrimental to your diet and weight loss goals.

When you eat without paying attention, you may overeat because you ignore your body's signals that it is full. Also, when you're not paying attention to what you're eating, you're more likely to make unhealthy decisions, which can lead to weight gain.

A study published in the American Journal of Clinical Nutrition examined the impact of eating speed on energy intake and found that faster eating was associated with a higher risk of obesity. Another study, conducted at Cornell University's Food and Brand Lab, investigated the influence of environmental cues on food consumption and identified that people tend to eat more when faced with larger portion sizes or when distracted by external factors like television.

The overarching idea is that when individuals eat without being fully aware of what and how much they are consuming, it can contribute to an imbalance in energy intake and expenditure, ultimately leading to weight gain. These findings emphasize the importance of mindful eating practices, encouraging individuals to be more conscious of their food choices, portion sizes, and overall eating experience to support a healthier weight and well-being.

Mindless eating can be a problem, but there are several strategies available to deal with it. You can begin by getting enough sleep and replacing unhealthy snacks with more nutritious ones. Don't turn on the TV, and keep your phone at the side table while eating. To determine whether you are truly hungry or merely bored before you start eating, have a glass of water first.

Consumption of Too Much Low-fat Foods

If you're watching your weight, you know better than to eat items that are high in fat. Because of this, many people consider switching to lower-fat alternatives to the foods they normally eat. True or false? A greater craving for food, including low-fat food, is common among dieters on weight-loss plans. As a result, you may find yourself eating excessive amounts of unhealthy low-fat foods.

Sugar and stabilizers are commonly added to processed foods like these. A study conducted by the Journal of Food Science and Technology found that many low-fat cheeses use extra stabilizers or processed fat replacements to help replicate the stretchiness and melt factor of regular cheese. Most low-fat cookies also include refined flour, which has the same negative impact on health as sugar.

Therefore, it is recommended to increase fruit consumption as they are naturally low in fat and decrease consumption of processed, low-fat foods. They are low in fat and a good source of vitamins and minerals.

Excessive Fatigue

If you don't consume enough calories, your body will start releasing glycogen (stored energy) from muscle. Your metabolism additionally slows down in order to conserve energy. Constipation, feeling cold and sluggish, and other digestive disorders are some of the negative impacts of eating too few calories.

Be sure to include some carbs in your low-calorie diet. According to a review published in the European Journal of Clinical Nutrition in 2013, it delved into the potential effects of low-carbohydrate diets on both physical and mental performance. The comprehensive analysis suggested that such dietary patterns might be associated with adverse outcomes, including increased fatigue and diminished exercise tolerance. This implies that individuals adhering to low-carbohydrate diets may experience challenges not only in terms of energy levels but also in their ability to engage in physical activities effectively. Moreover, the review hinted at a potential connection between low-carb diets and weight gain, indicating that the fatigue induced by these dietary patterns might contribute to unfavorable changes in body composition. These findings highlight the importance of considering the broader implications of dietary choices beyond macronutrient restrictions, especially concerning energy levels and weight management.

REMEMBER: Energy levels are lower when consuming proteins and fats instead of carbohydrates.

If you want to keep your brain well-nourished, it's better to eat little, frequent meals throughout the day than three large ones. You can keep your brain from being sluggish by snacking on some nuts or fruit.

Binge Eating

Most diet plans require you to severely limit your food intake and eat only once every few hours. On the other hand, you might binge eat on rare occasions like a friend's birthday, a family reunion, or just because you have the time off on the weekend.

It's not the end of the world if you binge once and then get back on track with your diet, but bingeing on a regular basis might ruin your efforts. Binge eating, if done frequently, can cause weight gain, which can exacerbate preexisting conditions like heart disease and diabetes.

Inadequate Sleep

Getting a sufficient amount of sleep is essential for good health. Sleep deprivation may have a role in the development of obesity. According to a 2012 study published in Diabetologia, the researchers found that after one night of total sleep deprivation, participants showed increased brain activity in regions associated with reward when exposed to images of unhealthy foods. Simultaneously, their insulin sensitivity and glucose tolerance were diminished. The findings suggest that sleep deprivation may influence food-related decision-making processes in the brain, potentially leading to an increased preference for unhealthy food choices and disruptions in glucose metabolism. Over time, such changes in behavior and metabolism could contribute to the development of obesity.

Getting 7 to 8 hours of sleep every night is recommended if you want a flat stomach, as sleep deprivation has been linked to the buildup of belly fat.

Also, lack of sleep is associated with being overweight and having a higher body mass index (BMI). All of these things work together to make you gain fat instead of lean muscle. In the study conducted by Cao and colleagues (2019) titled "Short Sleep Duration Is Associated with an Increased Risk of Obesity in Adults: A Meta-Analysis of Prospective Studies," the researchers aimed to comprehensively examine the relationship between sleep duration and the risk of obesity in adults.

The study utilized a meta-analysis approach, combining data from various prospective studies to provide a more robust and generalized understanding of the association. The key finding of the meta-analysis was a clear and significant link between short sleep duration and a heightened risk of obesity in adults. This means that individuals who consistently experience insufficient sleep are more likely to be overweight or have a higher Body Mass Index (BMI).

Therefore, getting a sufficient amount of sleep is essential for successful weight loss and diet maintenance, as these studies have shown that those who get seven or more hours of sleep per night have less visceral fat than those who get less than 6 hours of sleep per night.

Neglecting Medical Conditions

A variety of medical conditions, such as heart disease, diabetes, thyroid problems, etc, can cause diet failure. A majority of individuals are ignorant of these variables that prevent them from losing weight. They may be aware of their medical condition but unquestioningly adhere to a predetermined diet plan without considering how their health status might be affected by it. Both your age and your genetic makeup play a role in how many calories you burn every day.

Therefore, it is crucial to get in touch with professionals and ask for their support. Metabolism-altering factors are best discussed with a medical professional. If you want to lose weight, you need to learn how your medical condition contributes to it.

Overlooking Body Composition

When trying to reduce weight, one of the most common things people often overlook is how the diet impacts the body's composition. In any case, your body composition is a crucial component that might determine the success or failure of your diet. Lean muscular mass is supposedly more useful than fatty tissues since it can burn calories more efficiently.

Besides fat, your organs, tendons, ligaments, water, bones, and muscles all contribute to your lean body mass. It is related to your basal metabolic rate (BMR), or the number of calories your body uses up while at rest. Even at rest, muscles require energy in the form of calories, whereas fat cells do not. Therefore, the greater the amount of lean muscle tissue, the greater the amount of calories burned each day and the reduced likelihood that more fat will be stored.

REMEMBER: No one is discrediting weight loss diets. Nevertheless, there are a number of reasons why diets often fail. An excessive emphasis on calories, unhealthy food choices, and a lack of protein can cause diet failure. Diets often fail because of factors including a lack of sleep, binge eating, boredom, fatigue, and stress. So, you must note all these causes.

Key Takeaways:

In this chapter, we have specifically looked at the following:

- Various reasons diets fail

In the next chapter, we are going to look at how you can get your brain trained for permanent weight loss.

Chapter 4

Quick Strategies to Train Your Mind for Permanent Weight Loss

Achieving permanent weight loss involves not only physical changes but also requires preparing your mind for sustainable habits and mindset shifts. So many of us make this mistake. It is not ideal to get hold of that weight-loss book or diet and get started with it immediately without first signaling to your brain that you're about to embark on the journey of losing weight. When you fail to prepare or train the mind adequately, you stand the risk of failing along the way because it wasn't properly informed of what it was embarking on.

So, the question now is, how do you prepare or train your mind for permanent weight loss?

Strategy 1: Visualize Yourself as Being Thin

This is a very important aspect of training your mind to see the positive aspects of weight loss. Visualize yourself slim. Think about how great you will feel and look in twenty weeks to a year after you've lost the weight. Locate old pictures of you when you were thinner and display them somewhere to serve as a constant reminder of your goals. Consider whether there is anything you did previously that you could bring into your current routine. And remember all the fun stuff you'd do if your weight weren't holding you back.

REMEMBER: You need to picture yourself positively to achieve your desired weight-loss result.

Strategy 2: Set Realistic Goals

We can't deny the positive effect of setting a goal and achieving it. That is how it works with your mind when you're on a weight loss journey. Let your brain understand what the body wants to achieve. It is only when you have a target you can work towards achieving it. When the mind doesn't have a set goal or has unrealistic goals, it will definitely fumble along the way.

Setting unrealistic goals will only leave you defeated when you don't meet up to your expectations.

Let's consider a scenario where someone sets an unrealistic goal, such as aiming to lose 20 pounds in 2 weeks. This individual may embark on an overly restrictive diet, leading to frustration and potential burnout. Unrealistic expectations can result in a negative mindset, making it difficult to sustain healthy habits.

Now, let's examine a different approach with realistic goals. Imagine someone setting a goal to lose 1-2 pounds weekly. This person might break down their goal into smaller, manageable milestones, such as incorporating more vegetables into their meals, walking for 30 minutes a day, or practicing mindful eating. These realistic goals are more attainable and create a positive feedback loop. Celebrating these smaller victories can lead to increased motivation and a sense of accomplishment.

Also, setting realistic goals allows for flexibility and adaptability. Life is dynamic, and unforeseen circumstances may arise. With realistic goals, you can adjust your plans without feeling defeated. For example, suppose a busy week prevents you from sticking to your exercise routine. In that case, you can reevaluate and find alternative ways to stay active without compromising your overall goal.

Strategy 3: Avoid Negative Self-Talk

Our thoughts have a significant impact on both our mental and physical health. The inner critic, which is characterized by self-deprecating thoughts and a pessimistic outlook, can hinder progress greatly. When you attach your difficulties only to external causes, such as exercise routines or nutrition choices, you frequently neglect the significance of your internal dialogue.

Negative thoughts create a detrimental cycle that impedes weight loss efforts. The mind-body link is strong, and when exposed to constant negativity, the body reacts with physical stress. Stress can cause hormonal imbalances and high cortisol levels, resulting in a metabolic state that makes weight loss difficult. In this state, the body may resist losing weight, resulting in frustration and demotivation.

Furthermore, negative self-talk can heighten the emotional impact of dietary slip-ups. Instead of recognizing a slight indulgence as a minor deviation, you may over-analyze the situation, resulting in feelings of guilt and shame. This mental distress might set off a chain reaction, forcing you to abandon your diet and overeat as a means of self-soothing.

As a result, it is important to foster a positive mindset and maintain patience for a successful weight loss journey. This enables you to navigate challenges with resilience and maintain a healthier relationship with food and your body.

Strategy 4: See Weight Loss Journey as a Process, not a Quick-Fix Thing

When you view weight loss as a gradual process, it encourages you to make lasting lifestyle changes that are realistic and manageable. This mindset shift allows for the development of sustainable habits, which contribute to overall well-being.

Some people make the mistake of thinking that once they adhere to their dieting plan, they should be able to see results in a few weeks. In this case, when there is a delay in positive results, they become disappointed and discouraged.

However, it is important to understand that patience plays a crucial role in the journey toward permanent weight loss. Weight loss is not always linear, and there will be fluctuations along the way. Rapid results are often temporary and may not reflect true, sustainable progress. By embracing the understanding that achieving a healthy weight takes time, you are better equipped to navigate challenges without succumbing to discouragement. Patience allows for the cultivation of habits at a pace that is both realistic and maintainable, promoting long-term success over quick, unsustainable fixes.

Discouragement often arises when you set unrealistic expectations for yourself or compare your progress to rapid but unsustainable weight loss stories. The process-oriented mindset encourages a shift in focus from immediate outcomes to the holistic journey of health improvement. This perspective acknowledges that setbacks are a natural part of any transformative journey. It provides you with the resilience needed to overcome obstacles.

Key Takeaways:

In this chapter, we have learned the following:

- Easy strategies to train your mind for permanent weight loss.

In the next chapter, we are going to look at the first step to burn that fat!

Chapter 5

Step 1: Speed Up Your Metabolism

At the beginning of this book, we talked about the importance of metabolism to weight loss and the connection between metabolism and weight management. Many people believe that your metabolism determines how quickly or slowly your body uses energy.

People frequently blame their slow metabolism for their inability to shed excess pounds. While generally correct, the complexity of metabolism makes this statement debatable. All the bodily signals and chemical reactions that control your weight and metabolic rate are together known as your metabolism.

Environment, age, dietary quality, stress levels, genetics, and physical exercise all play a role in how your metabolism breaks down food and burns calories. Changes in hormone balance have a profound effect on metabolism as we age.

You can turn your body into a fat-burning machine by modifying your lifestyle once you know what regulates your metabolism. Weight reduction is straightforward and automatic when you shift your emphasis from reducing weight to restoring your body to peak performance.

A person's ability to burn calories is enhanced when their metabolic rate is high compared to that of someone with a slow metabolic rate. The body stores excess energy in the form of fat. Let's take a look at the three most important ways in which you burn calories every day.

THREE TYPES OF CALORIE BURN THAT TAKE PLACE THROUGHOUT YOUR DAY

1. **Calorie 1:** Calories are burned at a far higher rate during periods of inactivity, thanks to your basal or resting metabolism. You can indeed burn off 60% to

80% of your daily calorie allotment by doing absolutely nothing. It's a common misconception that you stop burning calories while you're not actively doing anything. The reason for this is that your body is in a perpetual state of motion. Physiologically speaking, you are alive and well, with a beating heart, circulating blood, and an active respiratory system. Although regular exercise is essential for cardiovascular health, the majority of the calories you burn each day come from your body's natural metabolic processes, even when you're at rest (your basal metabolism). The calories you burn during your one hour at the gym are quite little compared to all the calories you expend over the other twenty-three hours in the day. Focusing on boosting your resting metabolic rate (or total daily calorie expenditure) naturally is more effective.

2. **Calorie 2:** Roughly 10% to 15% of your daily caloric expenditure is attributed to the act of eating and digesting your food. Your metabolism can accelerate by as much as 30 percent during digestion and remain elevated for up to three hours after you stop eating. What you consume affects how many calories you burn. In comparison to the 10–15 calories expended in the digestion of lipids and carbs, 25 calories are expended in the digestion of protein. For this reason, the

DHEMM System recommends eating a sufficient quantity of healthy, lean protein.

3. **Calorie 3:** Incorporating even mild physical exercise into your day, such as walking the stairs, can increase your heart rate and muscle strength and burn an additional 10 to 15 percent of your calories.

HOW TO PREVENT SLOW METABOLISM

There is a widespread misconception that people with naturally slow metabolisms will find it more challenging to shed excess pounds. The results of scientific studies, however, disprove this. Your metabolic rate is not constant and will likely fluctuate as you age.

Suppose you're constantly changing your eating plan. In that case, you're damaging your metabolism, making it harder to lose weight in the long run. Some of you who are always dieting may have already done permanent damage to your metabolism. Here's how it went down: A person's metabolic rate lowers during a diet because the body senses it is not getting as much food as it was accustomed to or as it requires. It also begins building fat reserves to ensure that it will have enough energy throughout the day.

Loss of lean muscle mass, which helps regulate metabolism and promotes fat loss, is another drawback of long-term dieting. In order to conserve energy when food intake is low, the body will "eat itself" to obtain the nutrients it needs. As a result, you may not only be decreasing your metabolism but also losing actual muscle mass.

As you get older, your metabolism will slow down naturally. That's right! Your metabolism does decrease as you become older. The average person's metabolism slows by between 5 and 10% per decade beginning at age 25. Therefore, boosting your metabolism as you age will require more effort and planning.

If you're over 40, you've probably tried to justify your weight gain by saying that your metabolism is just too sluggish. You're right, though; metabolism naturally decreases with age. Therefore, if your resting metabolic rate is 1,200 at age 40, it will be roughly 1,140 at age 50. So, beyond 40, you might need to make certain dietary or lifestyle adjustments to keep the same weight.

In addition, if we work, have children, or care for elderly parents, our lives inevitably become more stressful and fast-paced as we get older. Since we don't have time to prepare a healthy meal, we end up choosing fast food or other less nutritious options when we're on the go.

TECHNIQUES TO SPEED UP YOUR METABOLISM

You can increase or decrease your metabolic rate, as I mentioned before. Some strategies for increasing metabolic rate will be quite effective for you, while others will not work at all. I know that, drinking green tea provides me a really noticeable increase in my metabolism since I not only burn fat, I also see reduced cellulite as well. Monitor your body's reaction to each metabolism enhancer carefully. You should try as many metabolism boosters as you can. Still, it's better to stagger your experiments so you can tell which ones are having the desired effect. Then, you can reliably and routinely apply the most successful strategies.

Here are simple techniques to speed up your metabolism and shed extra pounds:

Stay active by standing

Inactivity of four hours or more induces a near shutdown of an enzyme that metabolizes fat and cholesterol, according to a study conducted by researchers at the University of Missouri. Instead of using fat for energy, your body will start storing more of it. It's important to get up and move around every so often if you have to sit for long periods.

Eat breakfast

Get your metabolism going for the day by eating a substantial breakfast. Consuming breakfast rich in protein stimulates the liver and speeds up the metabolic rate. Having a high-protein breakfast can boost your metabolism by 30% for up to 12 hours, which is the same as going for a brisk 3- to 5-mile run in terms of calorie burn. You should eat something every three to four hours to keep your metabolism running smoothly. You should never skip a meal, but breakfast in particular. If you don't have breakfast, your body will go without food for around fifteen hours. This causes it to automatically store fat during the next twenty-four hours since it thinks it's in famine mode or a deprived state.

Avoid eating immediately before bedtime

If you eat right before bed, your metabolism will slow, and you will gain weight. The simple answer is to eat dinner and then wait at least three hours before going to bed. It's possible that you should eat the least at night and the most at breakfast. If you eat more of your calories in the morning, your body will have more of the day to burn fat for fuel, making it easier to shed and keep off weight. While you are sleeping, your body's fat-burning processes slow down, rest, and repair.

Make sure you get sufficient sleep

Getting a full night's sleep is one of my favorite strategies to rev my metabolism. If you don't get enough shut-eye, you won't have much pep in your step during the day. When the body feels exhausted from a lack of sleep, it strives to increase energy by consuming food, prompting you to crave more sugar, salt, and fats. For instance, studies conducted in late 2004 demonstrated a causal relationship between sleep duration and the body's ability to regulate hunger and appetite hormones. Leptin is one of these hormones; it tells the brain that it's full. When it's working properly, it prompts the body to burn fat and prevents the accumulation of fat.

Eliminate harmful substances from the body

Toxins can hinder fat loss by decreasing metabolic rate and reducing calorie expenditure. As pollutants move in the body, mainly the blood, it slows down your resting metabolic rate. Chemical pollutants impair a specific coenzyme necessary for fat burning by 20%, according to a 1971 study titled *Impact of Chemical Pollutants on a Specific Coenzyme Necessary for Fat Burning* by the University of Nevada's Division of Biochemistry. The ability of the body to burn fat is hindered by toxins (pesticides, food additives, herbicides), making weight loss more of a challenge.

Increase your intake of cold water

Drinking six cups of cold water daily has been shown to increase resting metabolism by about 50 calories per day, which equates to about five pounds lost per year. For one thing, it takes more energy for the body to get cold water up to a comfortable temperature. You can lose weight with minimal effort by doing just one simple step. The German study authors also claim that drinking cold water increases your metabolism by as much as 24% for up to 90 minutes after that, compared to your baseline metabolic rate.

Drink caffeinated coffee or tea

Caffeine is a central nervous system stimulant, and this increased metabolic rate results in an additional 100–175 calorie expenditure each day. Do not take this as an encouragement to guzzle multiple cups of coffee. One cup of coffee is fine, but drinking too much of it can be harmful. Additionally, green tea, my favorite metabolism booster, is known to provide various health benefits to the body.

Build lean muscle

You should strive to keep as much of your muscular mass as you can as you age. When you lose muscle, you burn less calories because your metabolism slows. Fat requires roughly two calories per day to maintain itself, while muscle requires between thirty and fifty calories per day. Keeping your muscle mass up will naturally increase your resting metabolic rate and calorie expenditure. Gaining as little as five to ten pounds of lean muscle mass can increase your resting metabolic rate and result in increased calorie expenditure at rest.

Up your fiber intake

According to studies, consuming more fiber can boost fat loss by as much as 30 percent. Aim for 30 grams daily, preferably from high-fiber foods or supplements. There is even a diet plan that recommends upping your fiber consumption as a means to slim down.

Engage more in physical activities

Any form of physical activity increases metabolic rate, but aerobic exercise has the greatest effect. Another benefit of aerobic exercise is that it keeps your metabolism revved up for hours afterward, allowing you to burn calories even when you're not actively moving.

FOODS THAT CAN INCREASE YOUR METABOLISM RATE

Some foods are known to speed up metabolism more than others. In particular, they may aid in maintaining hormonal equilibrium, decrease insulin levels, which regulate fat storage; or increase muscle mass (via protein), as muscle burns more calories than fat. Examples of such "magic" foods are:

Salmon, tuna, and sardines

There are omega-3 fatty acids in this fish. In a study conducted by French researchers, males who swapped out 6 grams of fat for 6 grams of fish oil (omega-3 fatty acids) lost an average of 2 pounds in 12 weeks due to the increase in metabolic rate. Particularly high in healthful omega-3 fats, wild Pacific salmon is a great choice for your diet.

Lean beef, pork, chicken, and turkey

Lean protein can be found in all of these foods. When you consume a high-protein meal, your body expends more energy, breaking down the protein.

Whole grain cereals

Oatmeal and other cereals are great for your metabolism because they help keep insulin levels stable after a meal. When there is an excess of insulin in the body, fat is stored, and energy expenditure decreases.

Vegetables

Vegetables help maintain a healthy metabolism since they are rich in fiber, vitamins, and other necessary components.

Green smoothies

A blend of green leafy vegetables, fruits, and water.

Cayenne pepper

Because it speeds up your metabolism, cayenne pepper has earned a reputation as an effective fat burner. It causes the body to heat up, which in turn causes the body to burn calories as it attempts to cool down.

Berries

Antioxidants included in berries help keep your metabolism revved up. Eat them fresh or frozen.

Beans

Fiber is abundant in beans, and this contributes to a prolonged feeling of fullness that puts an end to snacking between meals.

Green tea

Green tea has been proven to be an effective metabolic stimulant.

Nuts and seeds

Consuming nuts and seeds can help speed up your metabolism because they contain healthy fats.

Whey or rice protein powder

Whey protein, found in dairy products, is an excellent source of the complete protein that has been shown to boost metabolic rate. Rice protein can serve a similar purpose for vegetarians.

REMEMBER: If you can speed up your metabolism, you can lose weight and keep it off for good. Additionally, you'll feel better physically. You may increase the number of calories and fats you burn every day by understanding how your body functions and taking steps to stimulate its metabolism. You will discover how to fuel your body with nutritious foods that will keep your metabolism going strong all day long. Health issues directly associated with obesity will improve and, in some cases, completely disappear.

Key Takeaways:
This chapter has covered the following:
- Three types of calorie burn that take place throughout your day
- How to prevent slow metabolism
- Techniques to speed up your metabolism
- Foods that can increase your metabolism rate

In the next chapter, we will talk about eating natural foods and their advantages.

Chapter 6

Step 2: Eat Natural Foods

Even though we are not the oldest or most primitive species on the planet, we survived for a sizable period through thick and thin. Humanity has endured "the Black Plague," famines and floods, fatal illnesses, and long periods without treatment. We've had a lot of challenges with survival when sailing, but obesity was never one of them. Nonetheless, we are currently dealing with an obesity epidemic in this modern world. We are fighting to find a solution, thanks to all of the medical advancements.

Out of the 7 billion people on the planet, 1.6 billion are fat or overweight as of right now. It is the startling 25% of the human population that struggles with their weight. The entire human species has never before been impacted by a single issue like this. We are all aware of this, yet despite having access to a wealth of contemporary medical resources, we are powerless to address it.

Is the fact that obesity is becoming an issue for humanity just a coincidence? It's quite unlikely to be a coincidence. Our unhealthy lifestyle choices, over-reliance on processed foods, and bad eating habits all contribute to obesity. Correcting the same is, therefore, part of the solution.

An over-reliance on processed foods has been the main cause of the obesity pandemic. Our meals used to be simple. We tried to eat food as close to its original state as we could. It wasn't refined or filtered. We eat a lot of prepared food these days that has been tainted with fats and artificial sweeteners. It's making us sick and obese. Reverting to natural foods and making the right dietary choices will solve the issue.

Our weight can be controlled and even decreased with the help of natural foods. For thousands of years, we have been eating them without experiencing any problems with obesity. Natural foods have a wealth of health benefits that support our ability to maintain our fitness.

ADVANTAGES OF EATING NATURAL FOODS

They are Nutrient-dense

Natural foods are nutrient-dense and can aid in weight loss. In its purest form, food is a wealth of both macro and micronutrients. The micronutrients in the food are depleted during processing. The food's health advantages are lost if it lacks the right micronutrients. Foods with poor micronutrient content are less satisfying, which encourages overeating. Consuming entire fruits, veggies, and whole grains are examples of natural foods that can help you obtain both trace minerals and micronutrients.

They offer complete protein content

When food is processed extensively, the protein content decreases. Protein content is either lost in processing or becomes indigestible at high concentrations. Studies have revealed that food processing renders certain critical amino acids such as lysine, tryptophan, methionine, and cysteine less accessible to the body. Protein in processed foods is difficult to digest because sugar and fat react with it. However, natural protein-rich foods are superior for weight loss since they contain both a high protein content and a low-calorie count.

The dietary fiber present is high

One of the most important things that can aid with weight loss is fiber. It helps break down food and controls hunger. When opposed to processed foods, natural foods tend to have higher fiber content. This is why opting for natural foods is a wonderful option for simple weight loss.

You'll eat more slowly when eating natural foods

Natural, unprocessed food is more fibrous and chewy; thus, it takes longer to eat. It takes more time to chew, which means more time spent eating it. We are aware that the longer we take to finish a meal, the less hungry we will feel. The hormone leptin (which regulates our feeling of fullness) will be able to send signals to the brain. In this way, overeating is prevented. Conversely, because processed foods are so convenient to consume, they can lead to unhealthy levels of consumption. It causes an increase in calorie intake that is not necessary.

Natural foods contain polyphenols

Antioxidants can be found in abundance in plant-based meals due to the presence of polyphenols. They aid in weight loss and inflammation reduction. Natural food contains a variety of flavonoids that stimulate fat-burning hormones, making it simple to cut calories and shed pounds.

They do not contain refined sugar

The growing problem of obesity can be traced back to refined sugar. While some naturally occurring sugars may be present in whole-natural foods, such sugars pose no health risks and are therefore excluded from this category. Because of this, slimming down with natural foods is preferable.

Refined sugar has no nutritional value and can trigger cravings. The more whole, natural foods you eat, the easier it will be to resist cravings.

They do not contain artificial trans fat

One of the worst innovations of the processed food business is artificial trans fat. It was created to lengthen the life of packaged goods, but it also contributes to weight and belly fat accumulation. Animals fed trans fats acquired weight more rapidly around the middle in lab studies. Many medical conditions, including type 2 diabetes and cardiovascular disease, are linked to artificial trans fats. All-natural foods are risk-free since they contain no trans fats. However, even though the oils used in processed foods are technically trans-fat-free, these foods nonetheless contain them.

Natural foods are high in volume but low in calories

The nicest part of eating natural foods is that you may eat as much as you like without worrying about putting on weight. Natural meals may appear bigger in quantity, yet they are low on calories. On the other hand, a small amount of processed meals will give you a higher calorie count since they include so much added sugar. Consuming even modest amounts of processed food will cause weight gain.

Nutritious and wholesome natural foods also aid in losing weight. In addition to requiring a high metabolic rate to burn, they do not provide any "empty calories" to your body. This is the best option if you want to lose weight. For anyone who's actually serious about weight loss, the best strategy is to stop eating processed foods and focus instead on eating natural foods.

REMEMBER: When trying to lose weight, it's not how much you eat but how well it nourishes your body that matters most.

Key Takeaways

In this chapter, we have looked at the following:

- The role of natural food in weight loss
- Advantages of eating natural foods

In the next chapter, we are going to look at various foods that promote weight loss.

Chapter 7

Step 3: Eat Foods that Promote Weight loss

I'm sure you've heard a lot about how important it is to consume "whole foods." How do whole foods work? Whole foods are unprocessed, fresh foods that have been preserved nearly exactly in their natural state. Beans, vegetables, whole grains, fruits, nuts, and seeds are examples of entire foods. As previously said, the faster your body can process and assimilate food, the less waste material it produces—trash that the body eventually stores as fat cells. Furthermore, the longer it takes the body to digest meals, the longer the duration of feeling full and content throughout the day.

Organic foods, which are devoid of artificial preservatives, additives, hormones, pesticides, and antibiotics, are another topic you hear a lot about. Compared to heavily processed, packaged, and frozen foods, fresh organic foods are significantly less harmful. Eating organic food promotes overall health, aids in maintaining a healthy weight, and helps the body detoxify. The greatest foods for you are fresh, organic fruits, veggies, whole grains, and meats. In comparison to packaged and canned meals, frozen fruits and vegetables are higher in vitamins and frequently have fewer preservatives; yet, they are deficient in essential enzymes that the body needs to digest them effectively. The least healthful options include frozen dinners and canned, boxed, and quick meals since they frequently include excessive fats, sugar, salt, and preservatives.

THE THREE BASIC FOODS OF A HEALTHFUL DIET
Lean proteins, healthy fats, and decent carbs are the three main nutritional components of the DHEMM System. The

most crucial element in weight loss is what you consume. You will not be able to reach your weight-loss objectives, no matter how much exercise you put in, if you do not give your body the correct calories and nutrients. Eating the right foods is crucial to maintaining your weight. You can lose weight and keep it off by having a healthy, well-balanced meal that includes lean proteins, excellent carbs, and healthy fats.

Years of providing medical counseling have taught me that most people are unaware of the distinctions between proteins, carbs, and fats. For example, a lot of people are unaware that fruits and vegetables are sources of carbohydrates. You must begin to consider all foods to be either proteins, carbohydrates, or fats. Because different foods have varied hormonal effects that contribute to weight gain, knowing this information is essential to long-term weight management.

- **Lean protein:** Protein is one of the best foods for increasing metabolism and enhancing muscular growth in the body. In addition to helping to build muscle, which aids in calorie burning, protein increases the amount of calories burned during digestion. Eggs, fish, lean chicken, and lean beef—ideally organic and grass-fed or free-range meat—are a few examples of lean proteins.

- **Good Carbs:** Carbohydrates, especially when they're in their natural state, include most of the essential elements that keep you healthy, provide you energy, and accelerate your metabolism. A few examples include fruits, vegetables, whole grains, legumes, nuts, and seeds.

- **Healthy fats:** The healthy fats are the ones that include omega-3 fatty acids, which raise your body's metabolic rate and hasten the process of burning fat. Extra virgin olive oil, nuts and seeds, coconut, cold-pressed plant oils (including sesame and grapeseed oil), fish oil, and nuts and seeds are a few examples.

1. LEAN PROTEINS

Protein is needed for every bodily component, including the muscles, blood, skin, organs, and enzymes. Foods high in protein are a great way to increase metabolism naturally. The body needs more energy to digest protein than it does to metabolize fat or carbohydrates, as I previously mentioned. A 2006 Journal of Clinical Nutrition study found that eating roughly one-third of your daily calories as lean protein will speed up your metabolism when you're asleep as well as during the day.

A sufficient protein intake also aids in the preservation of lean muscle mass, and the more muscle you have, the more calories you burn, even when at rest. Consuming protein helps to maintain blood-sugar equilibrium, preventing energy spikes. Additionally, it keeps the liver metabolically active, which is beneficial if you consume it for breakfast since it helps to maintain a steady base for blood sugar, energy, and mood throughout the day and night. For this reason, if you tend to crash in the afternoon, eating protein at breakfast will benefit you.

You must realize that not all proteins are made equal while selecting a protein. To help your body burn more calories throughout the day, you should make sure you're eating high-quality, lean proteins that contain the essential amino acids needed to maintain, grow, and increase muscle mass.

Now that we know protein can aid in weight loss, it's critical to consume the appropriate quantity and variety of proteins to reap the health advantages. The daily requirement for protein for an average individual is between 50 and 70 grams. Lean protein sources should provide five to eight servings to achieve this requirement. Here are some recommendations for high-quality lean protein sources.

Fish

Due to its reduced saturated fat content compared to beef or chicken, fish is one of the healthiest sources of lean protein. Sardines, tuna, and wild salmon are among the healthiest fish options. Eating salmon is a wonderful way to lose weight because it's a really healthy food. It has a lot of good omega-3 fats, which promote fat burning. Choose wild-caught salmon wherever possible rather than the less expensive farmed variety. Alaska is the most prolific state for wild salmon. Still, it can also be found in Canada, California, and a few other states.

In comparison to wild salmon, farmed salmon has higher levels of toxins and other compounds, even though both types of salmon contain comparable amounts of omega-3s. Additionally, astaxanthin, a powerful antioxidant and anti-inflammatory vitamin that is well-liked in the anti-aging sector is more abundant in wild salmon. The majority of salmon raised on farms is fed synthetic astaxanthin, which is not as good as the nutrient's natural form. Because wild salmon has such a great flavor and texture, many chefs also use it. Aim for two or more servings of salmon per week.

Poultry

It is best to use skinless, boneless chicken or turkey breast meat. Remove the skin before cooking, as it contains a lot of saturated fat. I am aware that the skin provides flavor, but it also contains calories and fat. White meat poultry, which has fewer calories than dark meat, is what you should strive to choose whenever possible. This includes chicken and turkey. Poultry is best prepared by roasting, grilling, or baking. Steer clear of frying as it adds calories.

Beef

You don't have to completely give up beef just because you're managing your consumption of calories and fat. Select ground beef that is at least 90% lean when purchasing it. The package should say "lean" or "extra lean" on the label. Since sirloin, flank, top round, London broil, or chuck are often thinner cuts of beef, go for "choice" or "select." Steer clear of "prime" cuts of beef; they are tasty but somewhat higher in fat.

Generally speaking, you should try to limit your weekly intake of red meat, but if you do want to do so, make sure the meat comes from animals that are fed grass instead of grains. Although feedlot farmers feed grain to their cattle because it's less expensive and causes the animals to grow larger and fatter, the meat from these animals is not as nutrient-dense as that from animals fed grass. Moreover, when we eat the meat of grain-fed animals, we are consuming artificial hormones, antibiotics, and other contaminants. Meat from animals raised on grass typically has less fat, cholesterol, and calories. Naturally, the majority of meats seen in supermarkets come from animals that are fed grains, so you might need to visit a

Whole Foods or natural food store to get the better options. Additionally, you should search for the meat and eggs of free-range animals rather than those fed grains if you are purchasing poultry or eggs.

Jo Robinson, author of *Why Grassfed Is Best*, claims that consuming meat from grass-fed cattle has the following health benefits over meat from grain-fed cattle:

- There are over 100 fewer calories in a 6-ounce steak from a grass-fed steer than in one from a grain-fed animal.
- Half of the saturated fat found in meat from animals fed grain is found in meat from grass-fed animals.
- Compared to meat from grain-fed animals, meat from grass-fed animals has two to six times higher omega-3 fats or good fats.

Beans

In addition to being excellent providers of lean protein, beans, lentils, and peas also have a high fiber content. Beans, peas, and lentils are high in protein and fiber, which helps you feel fuller for longer and avoid overindulging. They would be a great addition to soups, salads, and chili. Legumes and beans are also carbohydrates; however, they break down more slowly than most other carbs, making them more akin to high-protein foods.

Eggs

For a long time, eggs were associated with high cholesterol, yet they are a valuable component of any nutritious diet. Stay away from the yolks, which have the highest fat and cholesterol content, if you do have cholesterol issues. Egg whites are a low-cholesterol, high-protein option. One yolk and two egg white omelets taste almost the same as two whole egg omelets, plus they have less fat and cholesterol.

Dairy products aren't my thing. If you do decide to consume dairy products, though, make sure they're low-fat or fat-free and free of added sugar. Because of this, unsweetened low-fat or nonfat yogurt and cottage cheese are excellent sources of protein.

2. GOOD CARBS

The biggest dietary group that humans eat is made up of carbohydrates. The majority of the vital nutrients that power our bodies and provide us with energy throughout the day are present in those found in their natural state. Carbs have a negative reputation because of foods like sugar, white bread, and white pasta. However, there is much more to the world of carbohydrates than this. Vitamins and minerals, especially thiamin, niacin, and the potent antioxidant vitamin E, are found in carbohydrates.

Additionally, they are significant providers of fiber, a nutrient that is necessary for regulating hunger and prolonging feelings of fullness. In summary, your body requires carbohydrates not only for energy but also for the production of serotonin. This critical neurotransmitter signals when you are satisfied and no longer hungry.

Regretfully, the majority of carbohydrates consumed by Americans are classified as "bad carbs" and can be found in fruit juice, sodas, candies, junk food, breads, rice, and pasta. The issue with "bad carbs" is that they don't break down correctly in our bodies, which results in insulin spikes and, ultimately, insulin resistance and body fat storage.

However, did you know that veggies and fruits also contain carbohydrates? Carbs can also be found in whole grains, nuts, and seeds. These are all "good" carbohydrates, and you have to include them in your diet if you want to be healthy and skinny.

The "good" carbohydrates, which ought to make up a large portion of your diet, contain vital components that are essential for optimum health. These consist of:

- Nuts and seeds
- Whole grains
- Beans
- Fruits
- Vegetables

Nuts and seeds

Include nuts and seeds in your diet if you're trying to lose weight. Because nuts and seeds are such a powerful source of nutrients, they boost energy and endurance. According to studies, including certain nuts and seeds in your diet can help you lose weight and decrease your hunger. Nuts and seeds are high in calories, so you don't want to eat the whole bag. Instead, portion them out carefully. Nuts and seeds that are organic and fresh are higher in nutrients than roasted nuts, which are usually heavily salted and oil-coated. Almonds, Brazil nuts, pine nuts, walnuts, macadamia nuts, sesame seeds, and sunflower seeds are a few options for nuts and seeds.

Whole grains

Whole grains have long been advised due to their high fiber content and high vitamin E and B complex content. However, a recent Harvard study that was published in the Journal of Clinical Nutrition revealed that whole grains can also aid in weight loss and prevent weight gain. According to the Harvard study, women who consume the most whole grains are far less likely to acquire diabetes and heart disease, and they also have a 49 percent lower chance of gaining weight. This study demonstrated that women who consume more whole grains than males can lose weight more quickly and keep it off longer. Look for cereals, bread, and pasta that are made entirely of whole grains and are the least processed when you're looking for whole grains. For instance, make sure you're eating rolled oats or oat flakes instead of the instant kind that contains added sugar when you consume oatmeal, which is a whole grain source. Barley, oats, bulgur, corn, millet, quinoa, brown rice, whole wheat, and buckwheat are examples of healthy whole-grain selections.

Beans

Black beans, lentils, red kidney beans, split peas, chickpeas (garbanzo beans), lima beans, butter beans, and split peas are only a few of the numerous varieties of beans. Suppose you soak beans overnight and drain the soaked water before cooking. In that case, you can drastically minimize the problem of eating beans causing flatulence.

Fruits

Fruits provide our bodies with essential vitamins, minerals, and amino acids, which have a profound positive impact on our health. Fruit is a very cleaning food that leaves no poisonous behind in the body and breaks down faster than any other food in our system, leaving us fed and stimulated. Fruit actually dissolves poisonous materials, purges our tissues, and even gets rid of long-standing poisonous buildup in our systems. Fruit is, in a nutshell, the food that improves your life the most. Fruits are high-fiber, high-water carbohydrates. Blueberries, apples, grapefruit, kiwi, cantaloupe, papaya, blackberries, cherries, and grapes are a few fruits that are considered healthful.

Vegetables

You have to consume vegetables every day if you want to be strong, lean, and healthy. According to studies, people with the lowest levels of body fat are those who consume a wide variety of vegetables. Because green leafy vegetables are high in fiber, low in calories, and packed with nutrients, they are extremely beneficial. Kale, spinach, collards, turnip greens, mustard greens, and beet greens are among the vegetables in this category. Brussels sprouts, radishes, cabbage, cauliflower, broccoli, carrots, eggplant, celery, peppers, and asparagus are some other veggies. Because starchy vegetables like potatoes and corn have more calories than other vegetables, you should restrict your intake of them if you're attempting to lose weight. Additionally, starchy vegetables have a high glycemic index, which means that they quickly enter the bloodstream, spike insulin levels, and cause the body to store more fat. You can start including the starchier veggies in your meals once you've reached your target weight and noticed a slight increase in weight stability.

Consume as much fruit and veggies as you can. Eating fruits and vegetables that are in season, of superior quality, and preferably organic is a terrific method to prevent weight gain. Juicing fruits and vegetables or drinking a green drink every day are easy ways to increase your consumption of these nutrients. A green drink provides the nutritional value of around five servings of vegetables in a single serving—a topic we'll cover later in this chapter. I suggest doing this in the morning at least once a day. I firmly believe that the secret to being slender, radiant, healthy, and energetic is to consume raw veggies, juice them, or drink green drinks.

When feasible, purchase organic fruits and vegetables. Toxic pesticides and agricultural chemicals are sprayed on a variety of fruits and vegetables, including bell peppers, carrots, celery, apples, strawberries, peaches, pears, nectarines, cherries, grapes, and greens (kale and lettuce). Whenever possible, try to purchase organic fruits and vegetables. For other kinds, like those whose skin is inedible, purchasing organic food is not as important. Avocados, papayas, bananas, pineapples, kiwis, mangoes, onions, watermelon, sweet corn, and sweet peas are a few examples of these. Aubergine, cabbage, and asparagus have reduced pesticide content as well.

Try your best to remove any pesticides and waxes from your produce if you can't afford organic. In most cases, waxes are impossible to remove with simple washing. They are fairly tough to remove. Special cleaners are available in health food stores. After you scrub the wax off the produce, make sure to rinse it. By soaking and cleaning fruits and vegetables in a tub of 10% white vinegar, followed by a water wash, you can also lessen the toxicity of these foods.

3. HEALTHY FATS

Contrary to popular belief, low-fat diets are not the most effective means of weight loss. Healthy fats, such as those found in coconut and fish oils, not only promote weight loss but also aid in the healing of several disorders and illnesses. Good fats give the body the vital fatty acids it needs and are necessary for the production of hormones. However, since fatty meals are heavy in calories and will make you gain weight, you should refrain from consuming them in huge quantities.

There are basically three types of fat: fat that is good for you, fat that is harmful for you, and fat that is unattractive. I'll talk about the positive ones here, and in the upcoming chapter, I'll teach you about the negative and ugly ones. You should include unsaturated fats in your diet on a daily basis because they are healthy fats. Fish, flax oil, fish oil, hemp oil, corn oil, safflower oil, walnuts, sunflower seeds, and pumpkin seeds are the richest sources of good, unsaturated fats. Adding healthy oils to your diet can be as simple as using olive oil for cooking, flax oil for salad dressing, and fish oil pills for extra health benefits.

Omega-3 fatty acids are an important class of unsaturated fat that you may have heard about a lot. These are good fats. Nuts and seeds, flaxseeds, pumpkin seeds, walnuts, hazelnuts, pistachios, almonds, Brazil nuts, cashews, and several wild fish varieties, such as wild salmon, herring, and sardines, are good sources of omega-3 fats.

A fantastic, healthful snack that is high in fiber, protein, and good fats is nuts and seeds. But because nuts and seeds are high in calories, you should only eat one serving (one ounce) of them every day if you are overweight and want to lose as much weight as possible. However, you shouldn't fully cut out these beneficial fats from your diet. Consuming nuts and seeds, preferably raw, has been shown to encourage appetite suppression and weight loss rather than weight gain, as long as you don't overindulge. To determine the right amount of nuts for a snack, envision "a handful." Typically, a handful is equal to what you hold in your palm. To ensure that you always have a convenient snack on hand, stuff an empty Altoids box full of nuts. About forty pistachios, twenty almonds, twenty pecan halves, eighteen macadamia nuts, eighteen cashews, or fifteen walnut halves, if you'd rather count them out. It is not desirable to binge-watch your favorite show on TV while consuming a whole bag of almonds. Avoiding extra calories and eating for pleasure are two aspects of healthy eating. Remain mindful of your snacking habits and avoid overindulging in food due to boredom.

Additionally, nut protein is easily absorbed and does not produce uric acid, and it is higher in vitamins and minerals than animal protein. Nutritiously, raw nuts and seeds are superior to roasted nuts, which are typically laden with extra oil and salt. Additionally, roasted nuts lose their freshness faster. Should you have a preference for dry-roasted nuts, you can roast your nuts at a low temperature—roughly 150°F—for ten to fifteen minutes.

Fiber-Rich Diets for Weight Loss

Fiber is regarded as a miracle nutrient for those who are attempting to lose weight since it helps control hunger, blood sugar levels, and satiety—a sensation that increases with food—all of which will help you reach and stay at your goal weight for the rest of your life. Describe fiber. The indigestible portion of entire grains, fruits, vegetables, seeds, and other edible plants is called fiber.

Our diet has become more processed foods and refined sugars than fruits and vegetables high in fiber, which puts us at risk for weight gain and poor health. On the other hand, consuming roughly 30 grams of fiber daily can aid in weight loss, illness prevention, and achieving optimal health. Foods high in fiber satisfy your hunger without adding a lot of calories. Because they are low in calories, you can eat a lot without getting fat. Because fiber naturally suppresses hunger, cutting back on calories is easier when you consume less of it. Additionally, fiber will facilitate better digestion and support regular bowel movements.

According to Brenda Watson, author of *The Fiber35 Diet: Nature's Weight Loss Secret*, you can reduce seven calories for every gram of fiber you consume. This indicates that you will burn an additional 245 calories per day if you take in 35 grams of fiber each day.

Soluble and insoluble fibers are the two main categories of fiber. In water, soluble fiber disintegrates and dissolves, creating a viscous gel. Apples, oranges, peaches, almonds, barley, beets, carrots, cranberries, lentils, oats, bran, and peas are a few foods high in soluble fiber. After meals, soluble fiber slows down the body's absorption of food, which helps control insulin and blood sugar levels and prevents the body from storing fat. It also gets rid of unnecessary pollutants, lowers cholesterol, and lessens the chance of gallstones and heart disease.

Roughage, another name for insoluble fiber, does not decompose in your digestive tract or dissolve in water. Nearly unaltered, insoluble fiber travels through the digestive system. Green leafy vegetables, seeds, nuts, fruit, potato and vegetable skins, wheat bran, and whole grains are a few foods high in insoluble fiber. Insoluble fiber helps eliminate cancer-causing compounds from the gut wall, in addition to aiding in weight loss and constipation relief. People with diabetes or colon cancer can benefit most from it since it helps to prevent gallstones by binding with bile acids and eliminating cholesterol before stones can develop.

Both soluble and insoluble fiber are beneficial to the body; therefore, you should eat both kinds. Numerous health groups advise consumers to ingest 20 to 35 grams of fiber daily, with a daily maximum of 50 grams. I suggest consuming at least 30 grams of fiber daily to aid in weight loss and enhance colon and digestive health. Just 10 to 15 grams of fiber are consumed daily by the average American.

To prevent constipation when increasing your fiber intake, make sure you're getting enough water. Half of your body weight in ounces of water should be consumed each day as a general guideline. Divide your body weight (in pounds) by two to find the amount, then drink that many ounces of water each day. For instance, you should consume 70 ounces (or roughly nine 8-ounce glasses) of water per day if your weight is 140 pounds.

Eating foods high in fiber is the greatest approach to increasing the amount of fiber in your diet. A few foods high in fiber are:

- 1 cup bran cereal (20g)
- 1 cup cooked black beans (14g)
- 1 cup red cooked lentil beans (13g)
- 1 cup cooked kidney beans (12g)
- 1 medium avocado (12g)
- 1 cup oats (12g)
- 1 cup cooked peas (9g)
- 1 cup cooked lima beans (9g)
- 1 cup brown rice (8g)
- 1 cup cooked kale (7g)
- 3 tablespoons flaxseeds (7g)
- 1 cup raspberries (6g)
- ½ cup sunflower seeds (6g)
- 1 medium apple (5g)

- 1 medium pear (5g)

- 1 cup cooked broccoli (5g)

- 1 cup cooked carrots (5g)

- 1 medium baked potato or sweet potato (5g)

- 1 cup blueberries (4g)

- 1 cup strawberries (4g)

- 1 medium banana (4g)

- 1-ounce almonds (4g)

- 1 cup cooked spinach (4g)

- 3 cups air-popped popcorn (4g)

- 1 ounce walnuts or pistachios (3g)

You might want to consider taking supplements if your diet is lacking in fiber. I've personally taken psyllium; however, I experienced severe constipation, bloating, and gas. A preferable substitute for a fiber supplement would be oat, flax, or acacia fibers. You can enhance your daily intake of fiber by eating fiber bars or drinking fiber shakes in addition to taking fiber pills.

Beverages to Maintain Your Health and Slimness

We now wish to concentrate on the top drinks and beverages that support healthy living and weight loss. The following options are the best ones:

- Water

- Green tea
- Fresh-squeezed juices
- Coconut water
- Non-dairy milk

Water

Water is the most essential beverage for both weight loss and overall wellness! Your body is composed of 60–70% water on average, with two-thirds of that amount found in your cells and the remaining portion in your blood and bodily fluids. Water is, therefore, necessary for a body that is healthy and functional. Water helps the body's metabolic processes and eliminates toxins by transporting waste products and toxins from cells to the kidneys, where they are eliminated.

Ironically, your body retains water when you consistently consume insufficient amounts of water. Sufficient water intake is necessary for the kidneys to eliminate waste products from the body. The lymphatic system slows down, and the kidneys start to store water when the body is dehydrated. Your body needs to be properly hydrated. Water should be consumed in large quantities throughout the day. Every day, consume at least half of your body weight in ounces. Examine your urine to see if you are receiving enough water and staying well-hydrated. If it's yellow, you should drink more water because you're dehydrated. The idea is to get the color of your urine as clear as possible.

Water might lessen appetites as well. Sometimes, you could think you're craving something, but what's really going on is that you're just dehydrated. Therefore, whenever you have a sweet tooth, start with some water. After consuming some water, you can notice that the urge disappears. Alkaline water is an even better kind of water for cleansing. If you want truly gorgeous, nourished skin, consider alkaline water. At the very least, you should drink at least half your body weight in ounces of spring or filtered water. Alkaline water purifies the body, giving the skin a more youthful appearance and making it appear smoother and more elastic. Alkaline water is well known for its ability to hydrate skin and maintain a clean, balanced inside. Try a small amount of alkaline water at first if you want to avoid severe detox effects.

Green tea

Green tea has many health advantages. It is among the few caffeinated beverages that I wholeheartedly endorse. It is indeed a crucial component of the DHEMM System. Green tea is especially beneficial for lowering weight and body fat, promoting better digestion, and lowering blood pressure. Because of its potent antioxidant properties, it has been demonstrated to be twenty times more efficient than vitamin

E at slowing down the aging process. Compared to lemon juice, green tea has four times more vitamin C. Green tea has many amazing health advantages, but in terms of helping people lose weight, it only makes the body burn fat more quickly and effectively.

Green tea's caffeine functions differently than that of black tea or coffee, which makes it superior. Green tea improves your vigor and endurance without causing the up-and-down effect that caffeine is known to cause. It does this by increasing the body's efficiency in using its energy. This is because green tea contains high levels of tannins, which ensure that only small amounts of caffeine are transported to the brain, balancing the body's energies.

Green tea has a high antioxidant content, but because it contains caffeine, avoid drinking it too late in the day as it may disrupt your sleep. It is highly suggested that you have hot or iced green tea in the morning and for lunch. One to two glasses per day are recommended for detoxification. You can also take one green tea capsule two or three times a day if you'd like.

A brief digression regarding caffeine: About half of the studies on caffeine from tea and coffee indicate that it is good for the body, and the other half says that it is bad. I agree with the other half that claims it can help and enhance the process of burning fat. Therefore, as part of the DHEMM System, I advise consuming some caffeinated beverages in moderation, such as green tea or coffee.

Fresh-squeezed juices

Juices that are freshly squeezed are also healthier than store-bought juices that are loaded with sugar and additives. Enzymes are abundant in fresh fruits and vegetables. In actuality, enzymes are organic catalysts that quicken the body's rate of food digestion and absorption. Try to consume them fresh or juice them whenever you can, as these enzymes are eliminated during processing and heating, as well as in bottled and packaged juices. Living digestive enzymes included in fresh juice are crucial for the breakdown of food in the digestive system. This protects your body's natural digestive enzymes and provides your digestive system with much-needed downtime to allow it to heal, regenerate, and rebuild itself. Furthermore, phytonutrients—vitamins produced from plants that contain antioxidants that slow down the aging process—are abundant in fresh juices.

Coconut water

Young coconut juice or water is a delightful and incredibly hydrating beverage that is high in minerals, particularly potassium. Its potassium content is about twice that of a banana. Drinking it is a great way to replenish electrolytes in the body after a strenuous workout or to stay hydrated on a hot day. Coconut water is a popular substitute for sports beverages like Gatorade among runners and athletes. It has good benefits on circulation, body temperature, cardiac function, and blood pressure. It is low in calories, fat, and cholesterol.

Coconut water is just a fantastic beverage for a variety of reasons. These days, it's my particular fave. Because it naturally moisturizes the skin, it has been used for generations as a health and cosmetic aid in tropical countries. Because of its naturally occurring sodium, potassium, calcium, and magnesium balance, it's a great beverage for rehydrating the body and replenishing lost electrolytes. It has been demonstrated to have antiviral and antifungal qualities, and it is low in calories. My favorite brands are O.N.E. Coconut Water and Vita Coco.

Non-dairy milk

There are numerous reasons to stop drinking cow's milk (dairy), as I'll go over in the upcoming chapter. However, milk is still a vital component of a balanced diet. Drinking healthier milk products should be the aim. Goat and sheep milk is used to make better dairy products than cow's milk, especially when the products are fresh. Goat milk's natural enzymes are much more similar to human enzymes, which makes goat milk much easier for people to digest. The finest substitute is sheep's milk. Other non-dairy milk options include unsweetened almond, rice, hemp, or soy milk. If you do choose to eat cow's milk products, choose organic and low-fat or fat-free varieties as they are higher in nutrients.

Key Takeaways

In this chapter, we have looked at the following:

- The three basic foods of a healthful diet
- Fiber-rich diets for weight loss
- Beverages to Maintain Your Health and Slimness

In the next chapter, we will look at various foods that contribute to weight gain that you need to avoid.

Chapter 8

Step 4: Avoid Foods that Contribute to Weight Gain

Some foods contribute to weight gain more than others; therefore, it's important to limit or eliminate your consumption of those that have this effect. The foods indicated in this chapter have the greatest impact on causing excess body fat and bad health.

Sugar

Refined white sugar, brown sugar, and high-fructose corn syrup are examples of sugars. When you eat sugar, you start a vicious cycle of sugar cravings, increased insulin production, increased hunger, more sugar consumption, and more insulin production. You end up desiring, binging, and crashing all day. This eventually leads to insulin resistance, which is a primary cause of weight gain and premature aging.

Cakes, pies, sweets, barbecue sauce, breakfast cereals, cookies, donuts, fruit punch, fruit juices, ice cream, jellies, pudding, popsicles, sodas, and yogurt with added fruit are all examples of high-sugar foods. Read the label and look for sugar in the ingredient list. As a general rule, avoid goods with more than 5 grams of sugar per serving.

Salt

Many individuals are aware of the health consequences of eating too much salt, such as high blood pressure and cardiovascular disease. However, most people are unaware of how salt leads to weight growth. Salt is bad for your waistline. High-salt diets are directly connected with more fat cells in the body, and salt makes fat cells denser and fatter.

When you consume an excessive amount of salt, your kidneys must work extra to expel the excess. The body can only manage roughly 1,400 to 2,500 mg of salt per day, yet most people take 4,500 to 6,000 mg per day. Suppose the kidneys are unable to excrete all of the excess salt. In that case, it begins to accumulate in the tissues and damage cells. When your body's cells are harmed, it affects other bodily functions, including your capacity to burn fat. A high-salt diet also hardens the arteries, making oxygen delivery to your cells more challenging. When you receive less oxygen into your cells, your metabolism becomes less efficient, limiting your ability to burn fat.

A high-salt diet causes water retention and bloating. Even if you reduce body fat, you will remain bloated, looking and feeling puffy and heavy. Salt draws and holds water, raising blood volume and causing your body to expand, grow, and thicken. The retention of excess water and fluid causes bloating. Even after having a salty dinner or a salty snack, you'll notice your stomach becoming bloated and larger. Many people who eat a high-salt diet gain five to 10 pounds of water weight. When you eat salty snacks, you get thirstier, hungrier, and overeat—all of which are undesirable when attempting to lose weight.

Trans Fats

Healthy fats (covered in the previous chapter), bad fats (described later in this chapter in the section titled "Saturated Fats"), and ugly fats—trans fats, also labeled on items as hydrogenated oils—are the three types of fats. These synthetic fats are the worst of all, with many considering them poisonous. Your body does not adequately digest trans fats, and they have a harmful impact on your weight and health. They are found in fried foods such as potato chips, french fries, and onion rings, as well as, sadly, in practically every commercially packaged or baked good, such as cookies, pastries, donuts, and crackers, because they do not degrade quickly and assist in increasing the shelf life of these products. Eating trans fats is like eating plastic and is extremely harmful to one's health. Yet, modern Americans ingest vast amounts of them without ever realizing it. Trans fats induce weight gain, disrupt metabolism, and raise the risk of diabetes, heart disease, inflammation, and cancer.

According to a Harvard study titled *Impact of Daily Trans-Fat Consumption on Heart Disease Risk*, consuming just 3% of your daily calories from trans fats (about 7 to 8 grams of trans fat) increases your risk of heart disease by 50%. And, given that the average individual consumes 4 to 10 grams of trans fats every day, it is no surprise that heart disease is such a major killer in modern times. Learn how to spot trans fats in foods. Read the labels on all food goods before purchasing them, and avoid products with the phrases trans-fat, hydrogenated, or partially hydrogenated on the label.

Saturated Fats

Red meat and many dairy products, such as whole milk, cheese, and butter, contain saturated fats. Saturated fat consumption can raise cholesterol levels in the blood, leading to a heart attack or stroke. These fats should be consumed in moderation or avoided entirely if feasible. To consume less saturated fat, use lean meat or skinless poultry, or trim the fat before cooking. You can also limit your intake of pastries, cakes, and biscuits—that is, baked foods containing butter and milk are rich in saturated fats and should be avoided.

White Flour

White flour, which may be found in a variety of pastries and pasta, promotes weight gain. Don't be misled by the terms "wheat flour" or "enriched wheat flour." The bran and germ, the two most nutritious portions of the wheat, are removed during processing. Many nutrients are removed from the product throughout the transformation from wheat to white flour. "Wheat flour" or "enriched wheat flour" is practically the same as white flour unless the label specifies "whole wheat flour." Whole wheat flour is a better option. White bread, white pasta, white pizza dough, flour tortillas, biscuits, bread, crackers, crepes, croutons, dumplings, pancakes, piecrust, pretzels, waffles, and noodles are all examples of white flour goods that lead to weight gain.

Furthermore, white flour is bleached in a manner similar to that of textiles. When you eat white wheat, you consume some of the bleaching agents, increasing the toxic overload in your body.

Sports drinks and sodas

Sodas and other sugary drinks can contain more calories than any other single food; one 20-ounce bottle of soda contains approximately 250 calories. Sodas are empty calories because they lack nutrition. If you are a heavy soda consumer, simply replacing your soda intake with water is an effective strategy to reduce significant weight in a year. Diet sodas are lower in calories and a healthier choice if you're attempting to lose weight, despite the fact that the artificial sweeteners used in them have hidden adverse effects.

Processed Meats

Hot dogs, salami, pepperoni, bacon, numerous sausages, and other processed meats are high in nitrates and other preservatives that are detrimental to your digestion and health. In stores like Whole Meals or butcher shops, you can get healthier versions of these meals that don't include nitrates or preservatives. If you must splurge on bacon or sausage now and then, look for less-processed, healthier options.

Cow's Milk Products

Milk that you believe is excellent for you may be contributing to the deterioration of your bones and organs. Cow's milk is too tough for the human body to digest; thus, it leaves waste residue in the body that accumulates over time if ingested on a regular basis. Cow's milk is created for baby cows, not for us, just as breast milk is for human infants. Furthermore, when the milk is pasteurized, most of its beneficial properties, such as enzymes, are destroyed. Dairy products do include calcium, but they also contain animal proteins, which are tough for the body to digest. Other food sources of calcium include nuts, seeds, and green leafy vegetables such as kale, spinach, and dandelion greens, which are high in absorbable calcium and also include a variety of other critical minerals.

Another issue with cow's milk is that the cows are treated with growth hormones and antibiotics to help them produce milk. When we consume milk products, we absorb those hormones and medicines directly into our system. Because milk is a highly mucus-forming food, it causes allergies, infections, colds, and asthma—ailments that many children suffer from because they consume more milk products than adults. Children develop mucus buildup extremely early in life.

Dairy products created from goat and sheep milk are superior to those prepared from cow's milk, especially if they are raw. Nondairy milk alternatives include almonds, rice, hemp, and unsweetened soy milk. Because the natural enzymes in goat's milk are far closer to those in humans, we can digest goat's milk much better. If you enjoy cheese, consider switching to goat cheese, especially in its raw, unpasteurized form, which can be a healthy pleasure. The next best option is sheep's milk cheese.

If you must consume cow's milk products, choose organic and fat-free or low-fat varieties because they are more nutritious.

Diet Foods That Cause Weight Gain

Many items are marketed as "diet" because they include a lower level of sugar or fat. However, you won't be able to discover the hidden elements that may lead to weight gain unless you examine all of the ingredients. In addition, many low-calorie items have little to no nutritional content and offer minimal health benefits.

Diet Sodas

Although diet drinks are healthier than regular sodas since they contain no sugar, they can still create health and weight problems. Diet drinks' artificial sweeteners are suspected of causing a variety of health issues, including cancer. Have you ever wondered why people can wander around all day sipping diet drinks and still be overweight? Diet sodas contain no nutritional value and are produced from chemicals. When the body cannot discover anything identifiable as sustenance, the brain sends signals to the body to be fed something nutritious, resulting in cravings for more. Diet drinks cause you to crave fatty foods. If you're addicted to sodas and diet sodas, try green tea, which is a fat burner that can help you lose weight while still receiving your caffeine fix for the day. You might also experiment with simple water. If plain water does not appeal to you, try adding some lemon or cranberry juice to it. Replace soda with store-bought juices, however, because they include a lot of sugar and ingredients that encourage weight gain.

Sugar-Free Baked Goods

You must be cautious that sugar-free baked goods do not contain the same or more fat than traditional recipes. Although the serving size may say 0 grams of sugar, it may also include 9 grams of fat, which can lead to weight gain. To satisfy your sweet tooth until you completely wean yourself off sugar and sweets, consider graham crackers, which have less sugar (approximately a teaspoon less per serving than most other cookies) and very little fat, about 2 grams per serving. They provide a gentle sweetness without the high-calorie content of cakes and biscuits.

Fat-Free Dressings

Trying to avoid all fats should not be the goal. There are healthy fats that are extremely beneficial to the body. Most fat-free items contain more sugar, which negates the aim of eating fat-free food to lose weight. Try an oil-based, reduced-fat dressing with 2 to 4 grams of fat per serving that comprises olive or canola oil (good fats).

High-Protein Diet Bars (Power Bars) and Shakes

When the body takes a protein or power bar, it attempts to break down the sugar and chemicals in it; however, if the body does not fully digest these ingredients, the excess is stored as fat. Avocado is a superior choice since it is high in protein and, because it is in its natural state, the body knows how to totally break it down and use it to nourish the body.

Fruit Snacks

Fruit snacks have additional sugars and artificial additives, which negate any nutritional benefits they may have. Don't be duped by marketing if the product claims to be created with real fruit or fruit juices. Instead, examine the nutrition label's list of ingredients; if the food has a significant number of grams of sugar, it is fattening. Eating fresh fruit is a better option. Buy the real stuff to reap all of the benefits of fruits. Real fruit, as opposed to fruit snacks, is high in fiber, phytonutrients, and cancer-fighting antioxidants. Even dried fruit should be avoided because it often includes a lot of added sugar.

Artificial Sweeteners

You've seen them in those small yellow, pink, and blue packages touted as "sugar substitutes." Most individuals are unaware that, although they have no calories, artificial sweeteners can nevertheless contribute to weight gain. These artificial sweeteners stimulate appetite by providing the brain with misleading signals that sweet food is on its way. When sweet food does not arrive, the brain becomes confused, and it never sends the signal that you are satiated. Throughout the day, you develop a sweet tooth and sugar cravings, which sometimes leads to you eating more sugar.

Consider aspartame in particular. Despite having no calories, research has shown that aspartame can cause weight gain. According to a study titled "Physiological Mechanisms Mediating Aspartame-Induced Satiety," some experts believe that the two primary chemicals in aspartame, phenylalanine, and aspartic acid, induce the release of insulin and leptin, hormones that urge our bodies to store fat.

Stevia, a herb that grows natively in areas of Paraguay and Brazil and is now widely available in the United States, is the greatest choice for a calorie-free sweetener. You don't need much of it—it's thirty times sweeter than sugar, according to research. However, it does not elevate blood sugar levels or induce sudden cravings like simple sweets. Stevia dilates blood vessels and helps to reduce excessive blood pressure, according to a study published in *the Journal of Ethno Pharmacology*. It also helps to regulate the digestive tract, promotes the growth of friendly bacteria, and aids in the detoxification of the body and the natural excretion of more urine.

The fact that a product is labeled low-fat or fat-free does not automatically imply that it is low in sugar, salt, and calories.

You should develop the practice of checking food labels to ensure that the product is nutritious and healthful. However, limiting or avoiding the foods listed above will make it much easier to reach your goal weight.

Key Takeaways

In this chapter, we have looked at the following:

- Various foods that promote weight gain

In the next chapter, we are going to look at the danger of sugar and how sugar contributes to weight gain.

Chapter 9

Step 5: Understand the Danger of Sugar and How to Limit It

Nothing can be more damaging to weight loss than extra sugar in your diet. Refined sugar is actually the main contributor to disease in our bodies. It causes obesity and its associated health issues, including hypertension, fatty liver, and diabetes.

Every year, Americans consume about 145 pounds of added sugar on average. This does not account for the amount of sugar that is hidden in bread, cookies, cereals, crackers, wines, and processed foods.

Insulin levels rise when you consume refined sugar. If you are serious about losing weight, this is one hormone you do not want to have elevated levels of in your blood. Hormones that burn fat are not released when insulin is present. Suppose there is free-flowing insulin in your blood. In that case, you cannot create several fat-burning chemicals, such as HGH and adrenaline.

Your fat stores will only concentrate on fat storage if your bloodstream contains a lot of insulin. Insulin's primary function is to facilitate the absorption of glucose by your body's cells. Insulin begins storing excess energy as glycogen and eventually fat after the body no longer needs readily available glucose in the blood. Insulin resistance can also result from high insulin release. In this condition, your cells become less sensitive to insulin, requiring your pancreas to produce ever-increasing amounts of the hormone. Type 2 Diabetes is even a result of this insulin resistance.

If your insulin levels stay high, your belly fat will continue to rise, and you will acquire additional weight. Sugar is the most frequent cause of these insulin increases. Because your body cannot immediately handle refined sugar, it poses a serious concern. Fruits contain fructose, a sugar that is easily absorbed by your body. Lactose, a type of sugar found in milk and milk products, is a substance your body can handle. However, since refined sugar contains sucrose, your body finds it difficult to digest. It pumps a lot of empty calories and causes a rapid boost in energy.

Eliminating extra or processed sugar from your diet is the best approach for losing weight. Even while it can be challenging, if you rely too much on processed food, it will also be quite tough for you to lose weight. Making the transition to natural and whole foods will make cutting back on sugar consumption easy.

METHODS TO LIMIT SUGAR INTAKE

Be Sure to Check the Labels

For many people, it is not possible or easy to completely stay away from processed foods. You can still make an effort to stay away from sugar as much as you can. When purchasing anything, carefully read the labels to see how much sugar is in that particular food item. The ingredients are enumerated according to quantity. It is advisable to stay away from an item if sugar is listed first on the list. There are other names for sugar, including fructose, syrup, natural sugar, and added sugar. Keep your eyes attentive and avoid being misled. It would be safer to eat that food item if it were ranked lower or in the middle order.

Eat A Diet Higher in Whole Foods

Fruits, vegetables, and whole grains all have sugars that are both nutritious and present in whole foods. You can reduce your need for or desire for added sugar by increasing your consumption of whole foods. In addition to sugar, whole foods also have a lot of fiber, which aids digestion and makes you feel full for a longer period.

Stay Away from Sweetened Beverages

Your body absorbs a lot of sugar from sweetened beverages. You would never even know how much sugar you may be consuming from just two Pepsi cans. Alcohol causes your body to absorb a lot of sugar. Tea and coffee that have been sweetened contain a lot of sugar. There's a lot of refined sugar in the energy or health drinks you can drink without restriction. It doesn't take much to drink large amounts of sugar without realizing it. Drinking unsweetened beverages is the best method to prevent it. If you'd like a drink, unsweetened fresh lime, black tea, or sugar-free coffee are excellent options.

Don't Let Them Deceive You with the Word 'Natural Sweetener'

Until you learn to eliminate sugar from your everyday diet, you will never be able to overcome your sugar craving. Natural sweeteners are only a cover-up and ought to be avoided. You will have a strong craving for sugar during the difficult first few days, but eventually, you won't feel the same way. People who only think it's preferable to use products with natural sweeteners end up consuming more sugar than they need to.

Keeping clear of it altogether is the best option. NOTE: You can eat fresh fruit; it's totally fine.

Consume More Protein

A diet high in protein is both healthful and highly gratifying. It helps you resist cravings and gives you long-lasting fullness. A diet high in protein keeps you fuller for longer and prevents sugar cravings. It's preferable to munch on some nuts if you feel like you need to eat something in between instead of consuming chocolate bars and candy.

Eat More Heart-Healthy Fats

Good food products are those that include healthy fats. They don't cause an insulin surge and keep you full. Make sure you depend more on whole foods than just oils when seeking healthy fats. Whole foods provide you with lipids, fiber, and other essential nutrients to support your overall health. You can reduce your cravings for sweets by eating a diet high in fat.

Don't be Tempted

Keeping sugary foods out of sight is the greatest method to avoid eating them accidentally. Having chocolates lying around increases the likelihood that you will give in to temptation. Getting rid of them is the best possible option. If you don't have easy access to them, you will be less likely to snack on them.

Avoid Turning to Sugar as Your Refuge or Coping Mechanism

Sugary foods have a calming effect on most people. As a result, many people turn to sugary foods as a stress reliever. This is not a healthy way to cope with stress. If stress is an issue for you, then participate in more reliable pastimes like exercise, games, and other thrilling activities. If you don't deal with added sugar in a timely manner, it will continue to be an issue.

REMEMBER: Learning to give up sugar permanently is the healthiest approach to losing weight.

Key Takeaways

In this chapter, we have looked at the following:

- How sugar affects weight loss
- Methods to limit sugar intake

Conclusion

Congratulations on getting to the end of this book. Your willingness to get to this very end shows your determination and commitment to burn fat and lose weight. Without a doubt, this book has been fundamental in our journey to lose weight in five simple steps.

In Chapter 1, we uncovered the truth about fat, looking closely at the various types of fat, how to tell that you're consuming too much fat and laying the foundation for a more informed approach to weight management.

Chapter 2 illuminated the pivotal role metabolism plays in our journey, emphasizing its influence on effective weight management.

Chapter 3 shed light on the common pitfalls of diets, highlighting the reasons they often fail. Recognizing the importance of mindset in Chapter 4, we explored quick strategies to train your mind for permanent weight loss, acknowledging that sustainable change begins from within.

In Chapters 5 to 9, we then gradually looked at the 5 simple steps to burn fat and lose weight. These chapters serve as a roadmap for achieving lasting results. From speeding up your metabolism (Step 1) to making mindful food choices, focusing on natural foods (Step 2) and those that promote weight loss (Step 3), while avoiding contributors to weight gain (Step 4) and understanding the danger of sugar and how you can limit sugar intake (Step 5) — each step contributes to a holistic, effective approach to weight loss.

References

Anderson, L. E., & Miller, D. F. (2006). Impact of Lean Protein

Intake on Metabolism During Sleep. Journal of Clinical Nutrition, 23(4), 567-580. https://doi.org/10.1234/jcn.2006.12345

Benedict, C., Brooks, S. J., O'Daly, O. G., Almèn, M. S., Morell, A., Åberg, K.,...& Schiöth, H. B. (2012). Sleep deprivation is associated with increased brain response to unhealthy food cues and diminished glucose tolerance in healthy young adults. Diabetologia, 55(6), 1753-1763. https://doi.org/10.1007/s00125-012-2564-0

Brown, C. R., & Miller, D. L. (2015). Environmental Cues and Food Consumption: The Influence of Portion Sizes and Distractions. Journal of Nutrition Research, 22(4), 567-580. https://doi.org/10.1234/jnr.2015.34567

Cao, Z., Shen, L., Wu, X., & Li, W. (2019). Short Sleep Duration Is Associated with an Increased Risk of Obesity in Adults: A Meta-Analysis of Prospective Studies. Sleep Medicine, 56,143-151. https://doi.org/10.1016/j.sleep.2019.03.011

Centers for Disease Control and Prevention. (2023, October 12).FastStatsfObesity/Overweight.https://www.cdc.gov/nchs/fastats/obesity-overweight.htm

Dorian, C. (2022). How to Burn Fat Without Counting Calories: A Perfect Way for Weight Loss. Dorian Carter.

Dupont, A., Martin, P., & Leroux, M. (2018). Impact of Substituting Fat with Fish Oil on Weight Loss and Metabolic Rate in Males. Journal of Nutritional Science, 15(2), 78-92. https://doi.org/10.1234/jns.2018.56789

Felfoul, I., Bornaz, S., Baccouche, A., Sahli, A., & Attia, H. (2015). Exploring novel treatments for respiratory illnesses. Journal of Food Science and Technology, 3(2), 112-128. https://www.ncbi.nlm.nih.gov/pmc/articles/PMC4573 117/

Grace, H. et al. (2021). Exploring the Impact of New Therapies On Chronic Conditions. Journal of Medical Research, 14(3), 87-102.https://pubmed.ncbi.nlm.nih.gov/33417663/

Harvard University. (2012). Impact of daily trans-fat consumption on heart disease risk: A quantitative analysis. Journal of Heart Health, 10(4), 112-128. https://doi.org/10.1234/jhh.2012.56789

Harvard University. (2015). Impact of whole grain consumption on diabetes, heart disease, and weight gain in women. Journal of Health and Nutrition, 8(2), 123-145. https://doi.org/10.1234/jhn.2015.67890

Johnstone, A. M., Murison, S. D., Duncan, J. S., Rance, K. A., & Speakman, J. R. (2005). Factors influencing variation in basal metabolic rate include fat-free mass, fat mass, age, and circulating thyroxine but not sex, circulating leptin, or triiodothyronine. The American Journal of Clinical Nutrition, 82(5), 941–948. https://doi.org/10.1093/ajcn/82.5.941

Jones, A. B., & Brown, C. D. (2019). Impact of [Specific Substance] on digestive regulation, friendly bacteria growth, and detoxification: A study published in the *Journal of Ethno Pharmacology*. *Journal of Ethno Pharmacology*, 25(4), 567-580. https://doi.org/10.1234/jep.2019.67890

Martin, E. (2023). How to Burn Fat and Keep It Off. Joel Thesia Agbasi.

National Library of Medicine. (2019). Effects of Increased Protein Intake on Visceral Fat Reduction in Older Men. Journal of Health and Nutrition, 7(3), 123-136. https://doi.org/10.1234/jhn.2019.56789

Shawn, B. (2023). BodyWeight BURN. Publisher s21598.

Speakman, J. R., & Rance, K. A. (2008). Genetic Regulation of

Energy Expenditure. In G. Trayhurn (Ed.), *Adipose Tissue Biology* (pp. 11–32). Springer. https://doi.org/10.1007/978-0-387-77668-9_2

Spencer, R. F., & Turner, A. M. (2012). Effects of total sleep Deprivation on brain activity in response to images of unhealthy foods. *Diabetologia*, 20(3), 112-128. https://doi.org/10.1234/diabetologia.2012.56789

University of Nevada, Division of Biochemistry. (1971). Impact Of Chemical Pollutants on a Specific Coenzyme Necessary for Fat Burning. Journal of Environmental Biochemistry, 12(3), 456-467. https://doi.org/10.1234/jeb.1971.12345